The **7** Naturopathic Secrets to Transform Your Health

The Path to Healing Through Natural Medicine

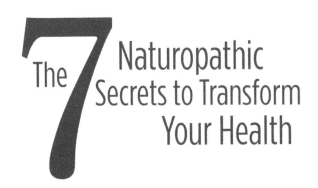

The 7 Naturopathic Secrets to Transform Your Health

The Path to Healing Through Natural Medicine

Dr. M. Samm Pryce

purposely
created
PUBLISHING

THE 7 NATUROPATHIC SECRETS TO TRANSFORM YOUR HEALTH
Published by Purposely Created Publishing Group™
Copyright © 2018 M. Samm Pryce

All rights reserved.

Printed in the United States of America
ISBN: 978-1-948400-02-2

Special discounts are available on bulk quantity purchases by book clubs, associations and special interest groups. For details email: sales@publishyourgift.com or call (888) 949-6228.

For information logon to:
www.PublishYourGift.com

DEDICATION

My mom and Aunt Sweet Pea have always said that I need to write a book and get my thoughts down on paper so that others can hear what they and my patients are privileged to hear. They have been supporting me before I even knew what that word meant. They encourage and counsel me strongly when they know that I am wrong. They are my rocks and my best of friends! Thank you, Mom "Butter Cup" and Aunt "Sweet Pea."

Without my husband, none of this would be possible. I am a tad old fashioned in the sense that I believe that the house and kids are my responsibility. Thank God my husband is not old fashioned. He cooks, cleans, bathes, and does everything and anything that is needed. During the writing of this book, he was no different, except that he did more. He never complained. He just said "do your thing" silently from the shadows. His love and support are why you all are getting this body of information and why I can be the best wife, mom, and doctor that God wants me to be. Thank you, Sean Pryce, my "Lovies."

To All My #VitalOnes

This book is for you! Let me start off by defining #VitalOnes. You should already know the definitions because you follow me on social media @DrSammND and you visit DrSammND. com daily, right? A #VitalOne is dedicated to health and wellness. They believe that there is a vital force—the body's inherent ability to heal itself—and the power of detoxing daily to maintain proper composition of blood and lymph and to decrease toxemia. #VitalOnes ask me questions about how to get healthy and stay healthy using natural medicine. I had no clue there were so many myths out there about natural medicine. Many of ya'll come see me in the office and haven't the slightest idea about the basics of natural medicine. So if you don't know what to use, when to use it, and how to use it, how are you going to feel great?

Crickets.

What you don't know might just be the answer to all your health problems! After reading this book, you will look at this natural medicine differently and hopefully know how to use it for both yourself and your family.

TABLE OF CONTENTS

Foreword by Dr. Peter D'Adamo 1

Preface 5

Introduction 7

The Naturopathic Approach to Health 9

The 7 Naturopathic Secrets 23

    1. Mindset 23

    2. Sleep 30

    3. Water 34

    4. Food 48

    5. Supplements 62

    6. Movement 89

    7. Detox 100

Summary 113

About the Author 115

FOREWORD

About a decade ago, I was a guest lecturer at the Southwest College of Naturopathic Medicine in Tempe, Arizona. During the lunch break, I was chatting with the college president, an old friend, and mentioned that I was interested in taking on a new graduate as an assistant. "I have just the person for you," he remarked. "I'll have her stop by later and introduce herself to you."

At the end of the day, a vivacious young woman came up to me and introduced herself as Dr. Samm Robinson. Within minutes of casual conversation, I could see right away that this person had a curiosity, dynamism, and enthusiasm about natural medicine that you do not find in all physicians. We hired her then and there.

Relocating to Connecticut, Samm threw herself into mechanicals of the clinic and mastering the work in personal nutrition that we are best known for. The patients loved her, and she showed a special skill in managing our therapeutic wing using time-honored naturopathic techniques to achieve cures when other more orthodox treatments failed.

After completing her residency, Samm moved out to the Midwest, and although separated by distance, we maintained our professional relationship and friendship. As I moved increasingly into bioinformatics software design, looking at genes and elements of the body's microbiome, Samm was right there, learning to master the intricacies of what are miraculous tools for precision medicine, but not within everyone's technical abilities.

Thus, it is with both pride and pleasure that I respond to her request that I contribute this foreword to her first book. What you are about to read, the journey you are about to begin, is in many ways a love letter to natural medicine; the belief that the body contains within itself the basic instinct to right wrongs, correct imbalances, and seek optimum performance. In the paradigm, the physician is not in the middle of the problem, where bad choices or insufficient information can only make things worse, but rather at the periphery, observing the tendencies and traits of the organism as a whole and helping to guide and channel recuperation and repair by supplying the necessary materials and procedural assistance.

How this is accomplished is amply detailed in the book, which is broken down into "seven vital secrets" (mindset, sleep, water, food, supplements, movement, and detoxification). In each section, you will find a treasure trove of prescriptive information that you can put to work right away. I know that you and your family will both benefit and enjoy this "vital roadmap" to health.

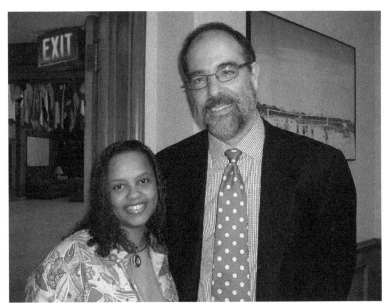

Dr. Peter D'Adamo and Me

Although I now only very occasionally write books for the consumer, I have had the experience of both great success and failure at the mass-market level. It is not easy to write simply and clearly about biological processes and disease patholo-gy, and I've met many brilliant physicians who never learned how to do it. Dr. Samm, on the other hand, seems naturally inclined to write in an easy-to-read, straightforward manner that is both engaging and inspiring. Much of the enthusiasm and dynamism that I remember in that young resident is amply displayed on the following pages.

Peter D'Adamo, ND, MIFHI
Distinguished Professor of Clinical Sciences
Director, Center of Excellence in Generative Medicine
University of Bridgeport
Bridgeport, Connecticut

PREFACE

My story is a long one. I have wanted to be a doctor for as long as I can remember, and I was on the right path to becoming a cardiac surgeon when God had other plans for me. In college, I became deathly ill, and no doctor could "fix" me. I had to wait and trust that my body would heal itself. I took this time to read books on alternative medicine and put some of the practices into motion to speed my recovery. I fell in love with the idea that my body could heal itself and that I could use natural elements to heal myself and others. I was absolutely entranced with learning all I could about this type of medical practice, and this is how I became a naturopathic physician.

This book is a combination of many of the clinical pearls that my patients get on any given day depending on what we are talking about and what questions that they have asked. Regardless of why a patient is coming to me or their chief complaint, it seems that at some point in their journey with me, we talk about these seven topics over and over and over again. I cannot emphasize them enough. This book serves as a written copy so that it can be read over and over and over again. These topics have blossomed into coherent thoughts and easy-to-follow concepts thanks to countless hours of teaching my patients. So, for that, I thank all my former and current patients!

I want to express my sincere gratitude to my mentors and fellow colleagues in the naturopathic profession. I want to specifically thank Dr. Peter D'Adamo for entrusting me with his life's work and teaching me everything that I know about the blood type diet. This knowledge has made me a better doctor and in turn improved the lives of many of my patients. Thanks to Dr. Letitia Dick-Kronenberg and Dr. Jared Zeff for exposing me and teaching me about food intolerances. Thanks to Dr. Tursha Hamilton for keeping me on track throughout this process. She has called and coached me through sections from the beginning. Last, but not least, thanks to Dr. Draion Burch for helping me find my purpose and making me finally write a book that has been long overdue. He believed in me and said I could do it!

INTRODUCTION

I hear complaints about fatigue, weight, pain, and the endless trips to this doctor and that doctor. The counter full of pills that people have to take to keep their body working. The unanswered questions that they leave with and the many other questions that these new pills conjure up. Stress, anxiety, and sleepless nights are not necessary if your body is in balance. Balancing your body is not simple, but it is doable if you have the right tools and you are willing to work on you.

Are you ready to be balanced?

The seven naturopathic secrets work independently of each other and synergistically. This means that you will get benefits even if you just apply one of the concepts. Of course, combined, you will get faster and more noticeable results.

Are you looking for results now?

I am going to teach you how to use things that you do on a daily basis to transform your illness into wellness. Things like what you eat, how you think, when to sleep and why are addressed. I will educate you on the use of water and movement and how these ssimple things can be used like medicine to heal your pain, help you lose weight, and decrease your stress. Adding in supplements like herbs, vitamins, minerals, amino acids, and homeopathy can help you enhance your overall well-being, stimulate your body's natural ability to heal itself, and give you more energy to do the things that you love to do with the people you love.

Does this sound like something you want to learn?

"Prevention is better than cure."
~ **Desiderius Erasmus**

Our bodies are amazing, and yours is no different. If we take care of it, nurture it, and listen to it, then we can have an amazing, vital life, free of disease and illness.

*"A **clever** person solves a problem.*
*A **wise** person avoids it."*
~ **Albert Einstein**

My goal in giving you these seven vital secrets is to help you prevent sickness, recognize the causes if it happens, and understand how to use the healing power of nature and your own body to heal yourself and your loved ones.

Don't you want to be both **clever** *and* **wise**?

THE NATUROPATHIC APPROACH TO HEALTH

Naturopathic medicine is not new. It is a very old way of practicing medicine. So let's start with a little history. Naturopathic medicine dates back thousands of years and combines the practices of many cultures: Indian (Ayurvedic), Chinese (Taoist), Greek (Hippocratic), Arabian, Egyptian, and European (monastic medicine) traditions. In the 1900s, when the practice was coined "naturopathy," it was determined that the profession included all natural methods of healing, including botanical medicines, nutritional therapy, physiotherapy, psychology (mind–body connection), homeopathy, and the manipulative therapies.

The first official naturopathic medicine class graduated in 1902 in New York. In 1908, The American Medical Association was going broke and literally was saved and bankrolled by Mr. John Rockefeller, who owned 90% of the standard petroleum making petroleum based pharmaceuticals. The Flexner Report of 1910 was commissioned by The American Medical Association (AMA), but to make it look objective, the report was said to be commissioned by John Rockefeller and Andrew Carnegie. The report was named after the author, Abraham Flexner, who was not a physician, scientist, or medical educator. The Flexner Report literally transformed the nature and process of medical education in America. It resulted in the elimination of proprietary schools (like naturopathic, osteopathic, and chiropractic) and established the biomedical model as the gold standard of medical training. It embraced "scientific knowledge and its advancement as the defining ethos of a modern physician."

Between 1910 and 1935, more than half of all American medical schools merged or closed based on this report by a single man. His aim was to decrease the number of graduating physicians, and he did so by only allowing men to attend medical school and closing all but two African American medical schools because he felt that blacks were inferior to whites and that they should only be treated by black physicians. Flexner felt that "modern medicine faced vigorous competition from several quarters, including osteopathic medicine, chiropractic medicine, electrotherapy, eclectic medicine, naturopathy, and homeopathy." [1] These schools survived for a while, but eventually all complied with Flexner's demands (osteopathic) or closed from lack of funding. Naturopathic medicine experienced a rapid and devastating decline in the 1940s and 1950s with all but one or two of its schools closing. Thus was

---

1   Stahnisch, Frank W.; Verhoef, Marja. "The Flexner Report of 1910 and Its Impact on Complementary and Alternative Medicine and Psychiatry in North America in the 20th Century." *Evidence-Based Complementary and Alternative Medicine.* 2012: 1–10. doi:10.1155/2012/647896.

born the evolution of pharmaceutical drugs, technological medicine, and the idea that drugs could eliminate all disease.

Naturopathic medicine is seeing a resurgence in popularity as modern-day drugs have several side effects and people just want more healthy and natural options. It combines empirical and clinical evidence with documented efficacy and adds scientific knowledge in areas such as biochemistry, nutrition, physiology, and botanical medico-pharmacology.

While the practice of naturopathic medicine is an art, all naturopathic physicians are guided by the same definition of our medicine, the philosophy behind it, and our guiding principles. These are unique to naturopathic medicine and set us apart from all other disciplines of medicine.

Naturopathic medicine as defined by The American Association of Naturopathic Physicians (AANP) is:

A distinct primary health care profession, emphasizing prevention, treatment, and optimal health through the use of therapeutic methods and substances that encourage individuals' inherent self-healing process. The practice of naturopathic medicine includes modern and traditional, scientific, and empirical methods. Naturopathic practice includes the following diagnostic and therapeutic modalities: clinical and laboratory diagnostic testing, nutritional medicine, botanical medicine, naturopathic physical medicine (including naturopathic manipulative therapy), public health measures, hygiene, counseling, minor surgery, homeopathy, acupuncture, prescription medication, intravenous and injection therapy, and naturopathic obstetrics (natural childbirth).

While there is a lengthy version of the definition of "naturopathic doctor," I like the definition that one of my mentors, Dr. Jared Zeff has penned: "A licensed primary care doctor who adheres to and practices in accordance with naturopathic principles and philosophies." When I am asked what a naturopathic physician is, my typical response is that I am an expert in natural medicine and bridge conventional and alternative medicine.

In order to really understand the concepts presented in this book, you will need to understand the principles and philosophies of naturopathic medicine as defined by the AANP.

Naturopathic Principles and Foundations of Practice:

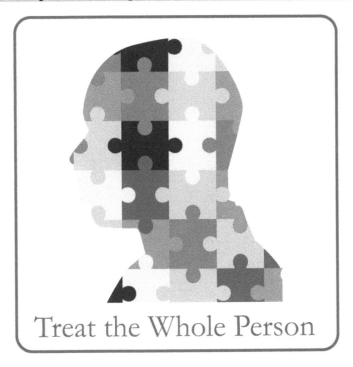

Treat the Whole Person

1. TOLLE TOTUM: TREAT THE WHOLE PERSON

The multiple factors in health and disease are considered while treating the whole person. Naturopathic physicians provide flexible treatment programs to meet individual health care needs.

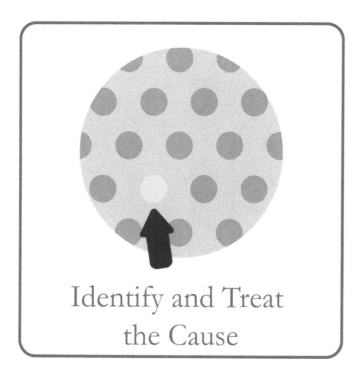

Identify and Treat
the Cause

2. TOLLE CAUSUM: DISCOVER AND TREAT
THE CAUSE, NOT JUST THE EFFECT

Naturopathic physicians seek and treat the underlying cause of a disease. Symptoms are viewed as expressions of the body's natural attempt to heal. The origin of disease is removed or treated so the patient can recover.

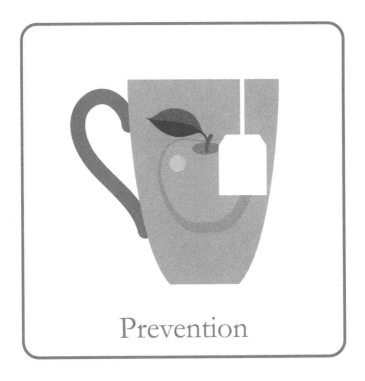

Prevention

3. PREVENTIR: PREVENTION IS THE BEST "CURE"

Naturopathic physicians are preventive medicine specialists. Naturopathic physicians assess patient risk factors and hereditary susceptibility and intervene appropriately to reduce risk and prevent illness. Prevention of disease is best accomplished through education and a lifestyle that supports health.

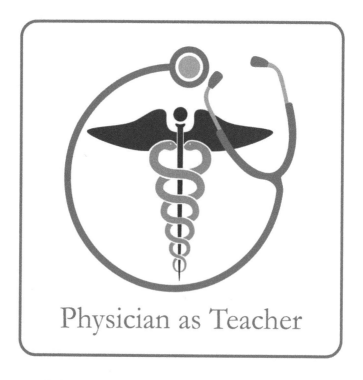

Physician as Teacher

4. DOCERE: THE PHYSICIAN IS A TEACHER

The word doctor comes from the Latin word docere, which means "to teach." The naturopathic physician's major role is to educate, empower, and motivate patients to take responsibility for their own health. Creating a healthy, cooperative relationship with the patient has a strong therapeutic value.

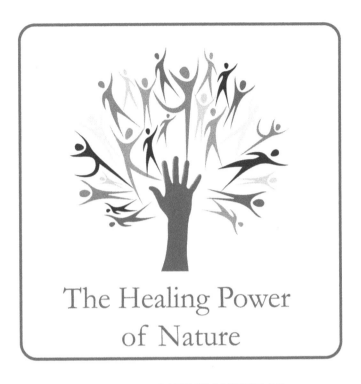

The Healing Power
of Nature

5. VIS MEDICATRIX NATURAE:
THE HEALING POWER OF NATURE

The human body possesses the inherent ability to restore health. The naturopathic physician's role is to facilitate this process with the aid of natural and nontoxic therapies.

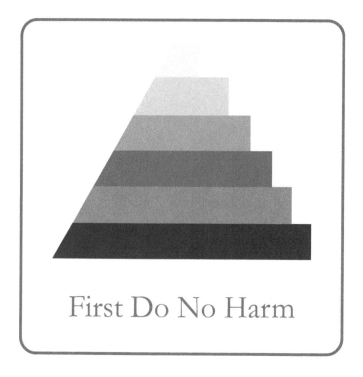

First Do No Harm

6. PRIMUM NON NOCERE: FIRST DO NO HARM

Naturopathic medicine uses therapies that are safe and effective. It aims to use the most natural, least invasive, and least toxic therapies possible.

It is based upon these principles that I really don't think that naturopathic medicine should be thought of as "alternative" at all, but rather primary. Your very first line of defense should be prevention. You should always be stimulating your body's natural healing force by first doing no harm, finding the cause, and treating your whole self while always learning more about your own body from your doctor. If and only if your body cannot rebalance itself through food, exercise, water, and rest should you move to therapies and natural supplements. If and only if your body cannot rebalance itself with therapies and natural supplements should you then try synthetic drugs and surgery as an "alternative."

When I (as a naturopathic physician) am treating a new patient, the above principles are used in my decision as to how to treat the person, but my initial thoughts are formed using our unique therapeutic order and how we think about illness in general.

Model of Healing: By Dr. Zeff

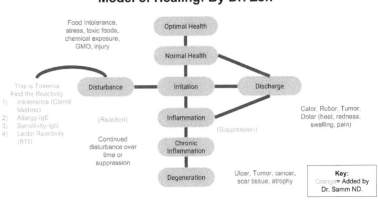

The current World Health Organization (WHO) definition of health, formulated in 1948, is "a state of complete physical, mental, and social well-being and not merely the absence of disease or infirmity." I read this simply to mean that all three aspects (physical, mental, and social/spiritual) need to be balanced and free of disease. Anything that alters the balance of one of these three states would be considered a disturbing factor, or what Lindlahr would call the causes of disease:

1. Abnormal composition of the blood and lymph

2. Accumulation of morbid matter: Toxemia

3. Decreased Vitality

Decreased vitality could be caused by such factors as stress, which would alter your mental state; dehydration or environmental toxins, which would alter your physical state; and negativity, which would alter your social/spiritual state. These reactions are acute and proper for a healthy individual. If the reaction does not occur, then we need to worry that the vital force is too weak to respond. Once the vital force or the body's innate ability to heal itself is done discharging and expelling the disturbing factor, then a state of normal health is regained. This cycle is called an acute reaction. If acute reactions are compounded one on top of the other with no discharge or detox, possibly due to a weakened vital force, then we find ourselves in a state of chronic reaction. Examples of this include anxiety from constant stress, headaches and achy joints from the untreated dehydration and environmental toxins, and depression from the imbalance of positivity to negativity.

In naturopathic medicine, we are identifying the exact disturbing factor so that we can remove it and discharge it from your body with proper nudging of your own body's ability to heal itself (the vital force) using the least invasive methods possible: lifestyle changes through diet, therapy, detox, and exercise.

Naturopathic physicians understand the healing process. We understand the healing order and that once the obstacle to cure is removed, the body's natural reaction to heal itself can occur. This is the reaction. Once we have a reaction, the expelling or discharging of the toxic substance can take place to restore normal health again.

If a chronic reaction is not reversed or is left unchecked and the disturbing factors are still at play, then we end up with degeneration. This is more difficult to treat and cure, but not impossible. The same thought process applies: find the disturbing factor, remove it, stimulate the body's vital force, and add supportive care such as diet, therapies, detox, and supplements.

The Thought Process

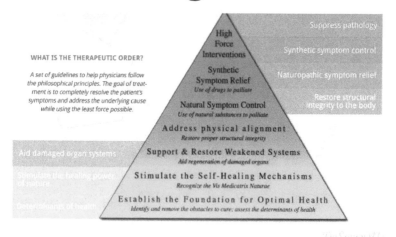

References:

Yanez, J. (2014). *Naturopathic Medicine Therapeutic Order Graphic.* Association of Accredited Naturopathic Medical Colleges. Adapted from:

Zeff, J. Snider, P. Myers, P. DeGrandpre, Z. (2013, January). A Hierarchy of Healing: The Therapeutic Order A Unifying Theory of Naturopathic Medicine. Retrieved from

Said differently, the foundation of naturopathic medicine is to determine the root cause of the illness (the disturbing factors), then stimulate the vital force to restore health by using physical medicine and natural supplements first. If all else fails, we turn to synthetic drugs and surgery.

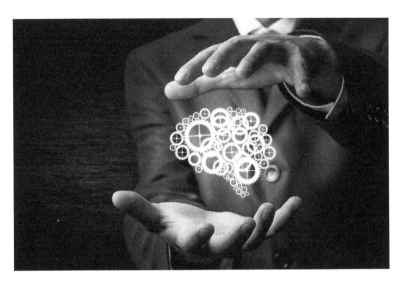

Mindset

There is something to be said for having a focus and intention that grounds you. Our thoughts often dictate our actions, which in turn can be helpful or harmful to our daily actions. Vital ones often hear me say "mind over matter." This means that whatever you focus on and believe to be to true *should* come to pass. Why? Because if you are really focused on it, you have no choice but to carry out all actions to make it happen. Let me explain further. We will use five vital secrets of mindset to get it done (improving health, wealth, or whatever you want).

The five vital secrets are intentions, affirmations, gratitude, meditation, and prayer.

A. Intentions

Intentions are ideas or plans for what you want to do. It is your determination or your plan to do a specific thing. You can have lots of intentions, but if you are laser-focused on a few, then it is easier to accomplish them. Think of them as your personal mission and vision statements. Here are some examples:

Overall and Broad Intentions:

I intend to be a loving and supportive partner to my loved one.

I intend to be patient and present as I parent my children.

I intend to live a clean and healthy life free of toxins and negativity.

Immediate and Specific Intentions:

I intend to ask my partner about their day **daily** and find ways to help.

I intend to help my child with their homework daily and listen to their concerns during dinner **daily**.

I intend eat a healthy breakfast **daily**.

B. Affirmations

Affirmations are statements or propositions that are declared to be true. They do not have to be true just yet. These are things that you want to be true—things that you are focusing on, meditating about, or praying about. Daily affirmations are powerful and can change your destiny. Many people write them on their mirror in their bedroom and say them while brushing their teeth. Some people do them as they are working out. They are great to include in your meditation practice.

Here are some examples:

I am cancer-free and healthy.

I am smart and beautiful.

I am employee of the month.

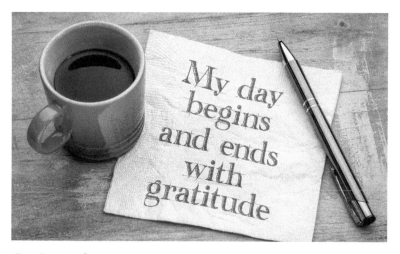

C. Gratitude

Gratitude is the key to success! We spend so much time focusing on the negative that we cannot even see our many blessings. If we focus on the positive and give thanks, we would not have any time left to think of the negative. Make giving gratitude a daily practice. Say "thank you" to someone for something that they did for you, or even someone else, whether what they did was in the present or the past. I give gratitude to my God at least twice daily in my prayers. You can give gratitude by having a journal where you write out your "thanks" or a gratitude jar where you write down your "thanks" and place them in the jar. The jar is fun because you could do weekly gratitudes and then open the jar on New Year's Eve to read them all. Being mindful of your blessings and acknowledging them makes you feel good and boosts your happy hormones!

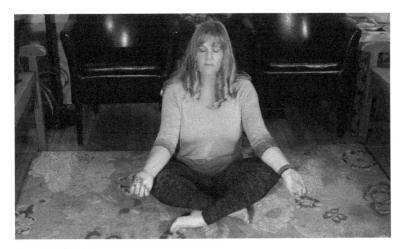

D. Meditation

There are many ways to meditate. Some consider prayer a form of meditation. The actual definition of meditation is thinking deeply or focusing one's mind for a period of time, in silence, for a purpose or as a method of relaxation. There is not a time limit on how long you meditate, and there's no right or wrong way to meditate. You do not have to be sitting on the floor with legs crossed or even have your eyes closed. I think that there is a false notion of there is a certain "way" to meditate. There is not. Individual meditation can be as simple as saying your affirmations or intentions repeatedly in your mind. It can be as complex as having someone take you through guided imagery. Meditation can be in a group or individual. The main goal is to deeply focus for the goal of relaxation.

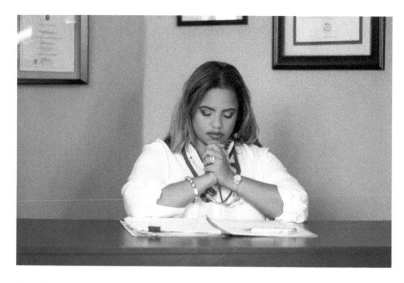

E. Prayer

As a Christian woman, prayer is how I start and end my day, and I know no other way. Before my feet hit the floor, I have said a prayer, which sets the tone for the day. I also end my day in prayer when my head hits the pillow and before I fall asleep. Don't tell anyone, but I often fall asleep as I am saying nighttime prayers, so I will wake up and start over. There is no right or wrong way to pray—it is personal and individual. My prayers are simple, and I follow a pattern that I will share with you. I use an acronym P.R.A.Y.

P. is for Praise. Praise the Lord and His name

Example: Dear Heavenly Father, I lift up Your name and give you all the praises.

R. is for Repentance (this is sincere regret or remorse)

Example: Father, please forgive me of my sins [you can be specific] as You forgive those who have sinned against me.

A. Is for Appreciation (counting our daily blessings)

Example: Father, thank you for all my many blessings. (Be specific.)

Y. Is for Yearning (the desires of your heart)

This is always the easiest. This actually (in my opinion) should be the most thoughtful. What we want is not always what is best for us. God knows what is best, and His timing is always perfect. If you keep this in mind, then you will never be disappointed.

Example: Father, You know the desires of my heart. I need peace in my heart and to be able to provide for my family. Please give me the knowledge and grace to find another job. Please open my eyes to see the open doors that You provide and give me the courage to walk through. Please give me patience for Your divine timing.

This, I believe, is more effective than Lord, I am stressed out and I need some money!

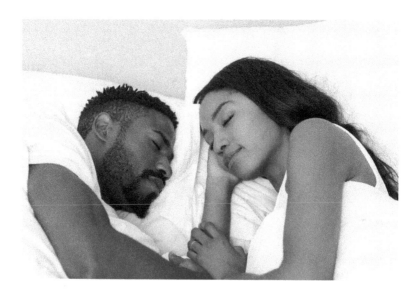

Sleep

It is no secret that sleep is my favorite pastime. I can go to faraway places and escape the day when I am asleep. It is one of my "go-tos" when anyone in my family is sick. My first recommendation is to go lie down and sleep. Why? Because the body heals itself when we are sleeping, and sometimes it just needs a little extra time. We are so busy nowadays that we rarely give the body the proper rest that it needs and deserves. Sleep is by far one of the most under-prescribed therapies, and in my opinion, one of the two most important things that we can do to increase quality of life.

A. Immune System

Our immune system is vital to our survival. It is the system that recognizes illness and alerts our defense mechanisms when necessary. When you have a cold, it is your immune system that alarms your body to either mount a fever to burn off the invader naturally or to secrete mucus to expel the invader. Our immune system can only function at its full capacity if the body is well rested, so sleep is vital to a robust immune system. They main controller of this power house of vital health is a hormone called melatonin.

B. Melatonin

Melatonin is the master hormone of the immune system, and it is produced naturally while we are sleeping. It is produced between the hours of 10pm and 2am. Let's think about this. It is the master hormone of the system that regulates and controls our health. It can be produced naturally without us having to take a pill or get surgery. This is true preventive medicine. Prevent yourself from becoming sick by allowing your body to produce the hormone to fight on our behalf. All you have to do is go to sleep on time! Wow!

C. Circadian Rhythms

I have had quite a few graveyard shift workers. Our bodies are not fooled just because they've gotten five to six hours of sleep at a time. The body wants to sleep in the dark and be awake and active in the day. This is called our circadian rhythm. Melatonin is produced in the dark. This is really hard to do when working the graveyard shift, even with blackout curtains. You cannot make it sunny while you are working at midnight. Your body needs some natural vitamin D from the sun. Graveyard shift workers often are at a higher risk for diabetes, heart attack, breast cancer, obesity, negative metabolic changes, depression, and decreased serotonin (feel-good hormone).

D. Hormones/Mood

Have you ever heard the saying "They woke up on the wrong side of the bed" ? This means that they are in a bad mood, so why talk about the bed? When you do not get enough sleep or rest, you become irritable, cranky, and moody. Think about a baby. When a baby starts fussing and is cranky, what are the three things you think of to assuage them? Diaper change, feeding time, or nap time. As that child gets older, they no longer need diapers, so we are left with two probable causes of the "fussiness" : hunger or fatigue. This is why people say, "It must be nap time." I am a huge advocate for adult nap time too. Google and some other progressive companies (usually abroad) are adopting this philosophy. They have found that productivity increases when employees get nap breaks, even if it is just a power nap. The brain needs a rest and re-set. Latin countries do a fiesta (lunch) and then a siesta (nap). They work long hours and are very productive because they give the body the rest, and specifically the sleep, that it deserves and needs.

E. Digestion

If you get nothing else out of this book, then you will get the importance of your digestive health. If you are not sleeping properly (not enough), then you are subject to your eating habits being off schedule and thus having digestive troubles, usually constipation. Constipation is the buildup of toxins in your body that cannot get out. This will cause skin issues such as acne. It also causes abdominal pain, headaches, and possible weight gain. These can all be avoided with proper rest.

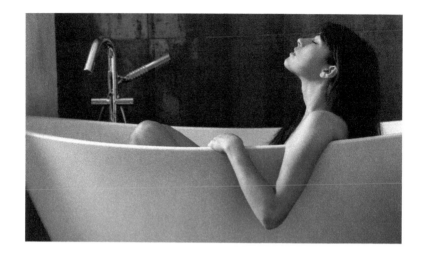

Water (Hydration and as a Therapy)

Just as air is essential to life, so is water. Our body is made up of 60% water because it is vital to life. You may have heard the advice to drink at least eight glasses of water daily. This is a good start, but to be more correct, you should drink closer to half your body weight in ounces daily. For example, if you weigh 140 pounds, then you should be drinking at least 70 ounces of water daily. In the elderly and very young, this may not be appropriate, so we can also use food, minerals, and vitamins that help with fluid balance to aid our hydration status. The main reasons why water is so important are that it:

a. Lubricates our joints to help use move pain free.

b. Controls body temperature through sweating.

c. Provides structural firmness to our cells and helps to make up blood, lymph, and waste (gastric secretions and urine).

A. Hydration (Internal)

There are both objective and subjective ways to assess our hydration status. I have two objective methods I use to test my hydration status quickly. The first is what I call the pinch test. It is testing the elasticity of your skin. It is very simple. If you are right handed, you use your thumb and index finger of your right hand to pinch the backside of your left hand. You pinch and then pull up. If the skin immediately goes back down, then I would consider you to be pretty well hydrated, but if it takes a second or two to go back down, then you are not properly hydrated.

The second method that I use incorporates what's called a Bio-Impedance Analysis (BIA) machine. The part of the machine that tells about hydration is the intracellular water and the extracellular water. I explain this as analogous to a grape and a raisin. They are the same fruit, but one is plump and hydrated, while the other is dehydrated. If we think of our cells as a grape, then what we should see on the BIA report is at least 60% intracellular (inside the cell) water and 40% extracellular (outside the cell) water. If those numbers are flip-flopped and there is more water outside the cells than inside, then you are really dehydrated. Sometimes I will see edema with this ratio.

The official definition of dehydration is "a harmful reduction in the amount of water in the body." Without doing any exercise, we lose about two cups of water. Drinking coffee, tea, and sodas actually make us lose even more water because they are considered diuretic in their properties and they pull water out of us. Most people think of dehydration only happening to athletes. This is not the case.

Another great way to easily tell if you are dehydrated is to check the color of your urine.

Dehydration can be fatal, and you should be able to recognize the signs:

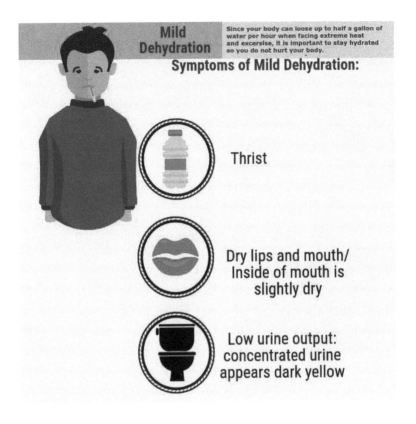

Mild Dehydration:

➡ Thirst

➡ Dry lips and mouth

➡ Inside of mouth is slightly dry

➡ Low urine output: concentrated urine appears dark yellow

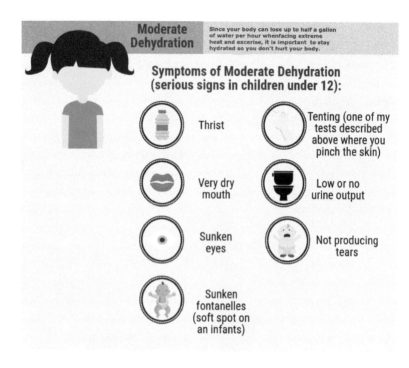

Moderate Dehydration: (these are serious signs in children under 12 years of age)

- ➡ Thirst

- ➡ Very dry mouth

- ➡ Sunken eyes

- ➡ Sunken fontanelles (soft spot on an infant's head)

- ➡ Tenting (one of my tests described above where you pinch the skin)

➔ Low or no urine output

➔ Not producing tears

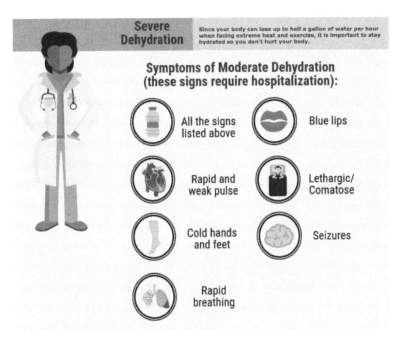

Severe Dehydration: (these signs require hospitalization)

➔ All the signs listed above

➔ Rapid and weak pulse

➔ Cold hands and feet

➔ Rapid breathing

- Blue lips

- Lethargic/comatose

- Seizures

Simple causes of dehydration may include:

- Excessive vomiting or diarrhea

- Excessive sweating regardless of the cause (endurance exercise, working outdoors, etc.)

- Fever

- Excessive urine output (uncontrolled diabetes, diuretic medication)

So, the million-dollar question is how do you hydrate yourself? I am sure many of you are saying drink water. Yes, this is partially correct. Water does hydrate, but proper hydration requires more than just the water. You can drink a gallon of spring water, reverse osmosis water, or distilled water and still not be properly hydrated. I can hear some of you saying Gatorade. Well, not quite. Proper hydration requires key electrolytes to be present and balanced.

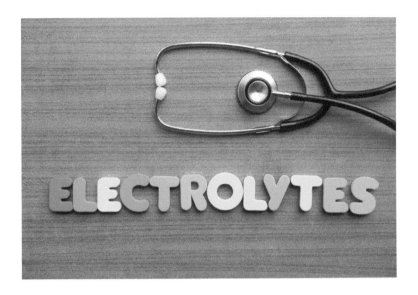

B. Electrolytes

Electrolytes are specific minerals that are essential to human health and cannot be substituted for anything else. I wrote about them in length in the supplement section of the book, but here is a reminder of their importance.

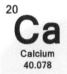

⊙ Calcium

Benefits: energy, nerves, bones/teeth, blood clotting, insomnia, menopause, obesity, blood pressure

Food sources: broccoli (increases your levels the fastest), turnip greens, dairy products (cheese milk, yogurt), nuts, canned salmon, sardines, seeds, leafy green vegetables (spinach), orange juice, cereals, oysters, rice beverages, soy, almonds, black-eyed pea, green peas

Symptoms if out of balance: hypertension, sleep issues, dental health issues, PMS, osteoporosis, kidney stones

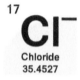

17
Cl⁻
Chloride
35.4527

⊙ Chloride

Benefits: One of the most important electrolytes in the blood. It helps maintain proper blood pressure and the pH of your body fluids. It also helps keep the amount of fluid inside and outside of your cells in balance.

Food sources: Seaweed, rye, tomatoes, lettuce, celery, olives, table salt, or sea salt

Symptoms if out of balance: vomiting, sweating or high fever (dehydration), diarrhea, kidney failure or disorders

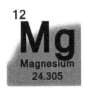

➲ Magnesium

Benefits: Enzyme activity and energy, prevents birth defects, muscle relaxer, sleep, constipation, anxiety and stress

Food sources: Dairy, fish, leafy greens, meat, molasses, seafood, seeds, soybeans, tomatoes, beet greens, broad beans, lima beans, artichokes, sweet potatoes, buckwheat flour, pumpkin seeds, peanuts, wheat flour, oat bran, barley, cornmeal, and chocolate

Symptoms if out of balance: Chronic fatigue, depression, insomnia, PMS, anxiety, insomnia, cramps, diabetes, heart attack, constipation, and migraines, nausea, irritability, muscle weakness, twitching, cardiac arrhythmias.

Overdose: Nausea, vomiting, low blood pressure, nervous system disorders

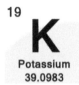

19
K
Potassium
39.0983

➔ Potassium

Benefits: high blood pressure, blood sugar regulation, boosts brain function, optimal nerve and brain function, optimal fluid balance

Food sources: fish (salmon), whole grains, citrus fruits, vegetables (broccoli, green beans), chicken, whole milk, fresh fruit juices (orange), almonds, nuts, lima beans, potatoes, avocados, bananas, coconut water, peanuts, bananas, oranges, sunflower seeds

Symptoms if out of balance: diabetes, mental fog, arthritis, kidney disorder, anxiety/stress, heart and kidney disorders, heart palpitations or irregular heartbeat, severe headaches, anemia, fatigue, nausea, anorexia, muscle weakness, irritability

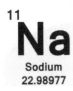

❷ Sodium

Benefits: water balance, prevents sunstroke, brain function, regulates sugar, skin

Food sources: apples, common salt, homemade soups, cabbage, egg yolks, pulses, bananas, carrots, baking powder and baking soda, turnips, leafy vegetables, dried peas

Symptoms if out of balance: muscle cramps, confusion, exhaustion, headache, diarrhea, weight loss, low blood pressure

Now, back to your comment or suggestion of Gatorade. Gatorade contains sugar, which defeats the purpose of hydration. The fact that a person with diabetes cannot drink a sports drink like this should be a red light for most. These sports drinks contain mainly if not only sodium and potassium as their choice of electrolytes added. The sodium content is astronomical, especially when most people get enough of this mineral in their daily SAD (Standard American Diet). The amount of other electrolytes when added is so negligible that it would not make a difference for true hydration. There are several waters on the market now that contain or have added electrolytes. My favorite thus far is Essentia. It contains sodium, potassium, magnesium, and calcium chloride. There are others, but you need to look on the label to see which electrolytes are added.

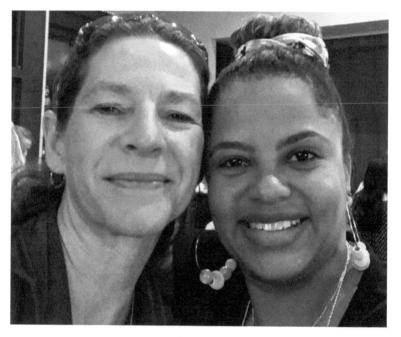

Dr. Letitia Dick-Kronenberg and Me

C. Constitutional hydrotherapy

Constitutional hydrotherapy is another way in which I use water in my practice. This is an old naturopathic therapy developed by Dr. Harold Dick and Dr. O.G. Carroll. Dr. Carroll called it a "constitutional" hydrotherapy because, "it changes the very constitution of each cell." He taught this method one or two others, and it has since been passed down through the generations. I was taught the therapy at naturopathic medical school. I used it heavily in my residency in Connecticut with Dr. Peter D'Adamo and then was blessed to be taught by Dr. Dick's daughter to improve my skills later in my career. The therapy is simple in its application but powerful in its results. You use alternating hot and cold towels in a very strategic order along with surging sine waves placed on certain areas of the body to elicit a therapeutic response from the body. This therapy is one of the cornerstones of my practice. It has been credited with increasing vitality, decreasing pain, decreasing body fat, increasing T3, T4 and T7 (energy creators related to metabolism), resolving constipation, and decreasing 15 points in arterial pressure.

D. Digestion/Poop

"Here she goes again." I hear you saying it. Yes, I will say it over and over again. You must poop! The only way you are going to poop or do it effectively is to have proper digestion. You must be able to digest your foods and metabolize them properly. Hydration allows for a smooth passage of the waste to leave your body without pain (constipation free). Proper water intake softens the waste water. Most people think that constipation is just measured in the number of times that you go per day or week, but it is also measured in the amount eliminated and whether or not it is painful. Small balls that are painful is considered constipation. This is remedied by proper hydration.

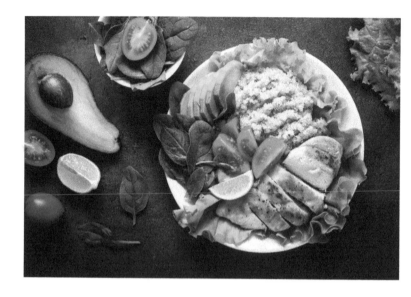

Food

This is one of my favorite topics because it is so vital to our overall health. We are what we eat, literally. Hippocrates (the founder of medicine as we know it) coined the phrase "Let food be thy medicine and medicine be thy food." I have always been fascinated by this, and so it is a huge part of how I manage and heal my patients quickly without conventional medication.

A. Blood Type Diet

The Blood Type Diet is one of my secret weapons for living a long and vital life. I have my mentor Dr. Peter D'Adamo to thank for teaching me all that I know on this subject and being able to share it with you and all of my patients. We all must eat food to survive, so why not eat those foods that are specifically going to act as medicine to keep us healthy and decrease inflammation? This is so much easier than popping pills daily and having to do surgery. Just eat according to your blood type. Why? Because this is how your ancestors ate, and according to your DNA, how to get the most bang for your buck when it comes to your food choices.

I am sure you have wondered, "Why did the Atkins diet work for me and not my friend?" or "Why is my friend who has switched to a plant-based diet (vegetarian) lost weight but when I tried I didn't and I ended up sick?" Great questions! The answer is because you all have different blood types, and one diet solution does not work for all. By breaking it down into blood type–specific foods and categorizing them as beneficial (medicinal), avoid (causes inflammation), or neutral (neither good nor bad, so can be eaten in moderation), we get a more customized approach to how your eating should be based on genetics. Without getting into too much detail, we can then use this knowledge to further help to express genes by turning them either on or off using these food choices. This is called epigenetics using nutrigenomics. This is a powerful, scientifically studied way in which food can be used as medicine using what we know about lectins (proteins). So let me tell you about the four different blood types and share a few secrets with you.

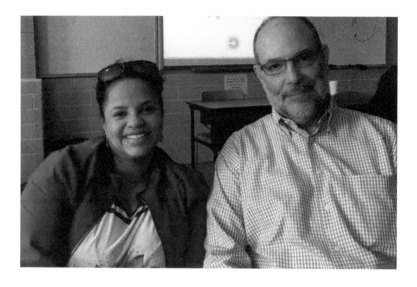

Dr. Peter D'Adamo and Me

B. Blood Type O

This blood type is the oldest. It comes from the hunters back when the earth was covered in ice and we needed to hunt for our food. Since they hunted and ate mainly meat, their stomachs were adapted with a high amount of hydrochloric acid (the acid needed to break down meat). This blood type should be meat eaters. See the chart below/on the following pages for more information.

TYPE O (THE HUNTER– STRONG, SELF RELIANT, LEADER)

STRENGTHS	WEAKNESS	MEDICAL RISKS
Hardy digestive tract Strong immune sys Natural defenses against infections Designed for efficient metabolism & preservation of nutrients	Intolerant to new dietary and environmental conditions Immune sys can be overactive and attack itself	Blood Clotting Disorders Inflammatory Disease-Arthritis Low Thyroid production Ulcers Allergies
DIET PROFILE	**WEIGHT LOSS KEY**	**SUPPLEMENTS**
High Protein: Meat Eaters Meat, Fish, Vegetables, Fruit Limited: Grains, Beans, Legumes	**AVOID** Wheat, corn, kidney beans, navy beans, lentil, cabbage, brussel sprouts, cauliflower, mustard greens **AIDS** Kelp, Seafood, salt, liver, red meat, kale, spinach, broccoli	Vit B, Vit K, Calcium, Iodine, Licorice, Kelp

C. Blood Type A

As the ice melted, we became more of an agrarian society (farming/gathering). We did not hunt as much, and thus our stomachs did not need as much acid, so it did not produce as much. This acid is needed to break down red meat specifically, so without it, this blood type cannot break it down properly. If you are this blood type, you should be a vegetarian and get most of your protein from beans and legumes. Just because you are a vegetarian does not mean that you should not have the proper amount of protein. I have seen this go horribly wrong. I see patients who have attempted to go on a vegetarian diet or lifestyle change, but in actuality they are now carbotarians (a made-up word for those people who mainly eat carbs) and add in a few veggies. There is a tricky balance, and protein is a must in all diets.

TYPE A (THE CULTIVATOR-SETTLED, COOPERATIVE, ORDERLY, ARTISTIC VISIONARY)		
STRENGTHS	**WEAKNESS**	**MEDICAL RISKS**
Adapts well to dietary and environmental changes

Immune sys preserves and metabolizes nutrients more easily | Sensitive Digestive Tract

Vulnerable immune system, open to microbial invasion | Heart Disease

Cancer

Anemia

Liver/Gallbladder disorders

Type 1 Diabetes |
| **DIET PROFILE** | **WEIGHT LOSS KEY** | **SUPPLEMENTS** |
| Vegetarian

Vegetables, tofu, seafood, grains, beans, legumes, fruit | **AVOID**

Meat, dairy, kidney beans, lima beans, wheat

AIDS

Vegetable Oils, soy foods, pineapple | Vit B12, folic Acid, Vit C, Vit E, Hawthorn, Echinacea, Quercetin, Milk Thistle |

D. Blood Type B

As we continue through our evolution journey, we then adapted into blood type B. Some say that B is for best. There is no best blood type. If you have this blood type, you have some oddities in your diet, in that you do not do well at all with corn, chicken, and soy, all thought to be healthy food choices, but not at all for you. I have seen this over and over again with my patients with migraine headaches. My first question for a patient who comes in complaining of migraine headaches is "What is your blood type?" If they are a blood type B, nine times out of ten, they are addicted to one of the three food items (chicken, corn, or soy). I suggest removing this from the diet for at least two weeks just to test it out, and it never fails. The headaches go away!

TYPE B (THE NOMAD-BALANCED, FLEXIBLE, CREATIVE)

STRENGTHS	WEAKNESS	MEDICAL RISKS
Strong Immune sys	No natural weakness BUT imbalance causes tendency toward auto-immune breakdowns and rare viruses	Type 1 Diabetes Chronic Fatigue Syndrome Autoimmune disorders- Lupus, ALS, MS
DIET PROFILE	**WEIGHT LOSS KEY**	**SUPPLEMENTS**
Balanced Omnivore Meat- (NO chicken) Dairy, Grains, Beans, Legumes, vegetables, Fruit	**AVOID** Corn, Lentils, Peanuts, Sesame seeds, Buckwheat, Wheat **AIDS** Greens, Eggs, Venison, Liver, Licorice, Tea	Magnesium Licorice Ginko Lecithin

E. Blood Type AB

My bonus son has this blood type, and it is very interesting. It is the only one that did not come from evolution, but more of a mingling of type A and type B (I am still trying to figure this out myself). Since both blood type A and Blood Type B are dominant, blood type AB shares characteristics of both blood type A and B (the good and the bad).

TYPE AB (THE ENIGMA- RARE, CHARISMATIC, MYSTERIOUS)		
STRENGTHS	**WEAKNESS**	**MEDICAL RISKS**
Designed for modern conditions Highly tolerant immune system Combines benefits of Type A and Type B	Sensitive digestive tract Tendency for over-tolerant immune system allowing microbial invasion Vulnerable to A-like and B-like medical conditions	Heart Disease Cancer Anemia
DIET PROFILE	**WEIGHT LOSS KEY**	**SUPPLEMENTS**
Mixed diet in moderation Meat, seafood, dairy, tofu, beans, legumes, grains, vegetable, fruit	**AVOID** Red meat, Kidney beans, Lima beans, Seeds, Corn, Buckwheat **AIDS** Tofu, Seafood, Dairy, Greens, Kelp, Pineapple	Vit C Hawthorn Echinacea Valerian Quercetin Milk Thistle

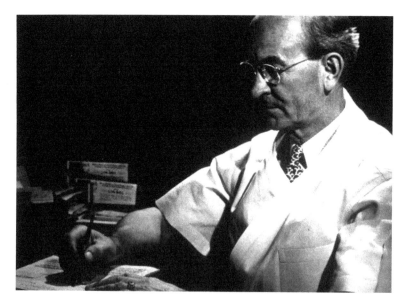

O.G. Carroll

THE CARROLL METHOD

This is my newest secret for healing my patients. I feel like this is one of the best-kept secrets because not a lot of people know about it. It is an over-100-year-old naturopathic way of looking at how your body digests certain foods and whether or not you can metabolize certain foods properly. No other school of medicine but naturopathic medicine can do this. It is not a test, but a way of honing into a person's vital force and seeing if it was designed to accept or discard certain foods. Through years of practice and thousands and thousands of case studies, Dr. Otis G. Carroll mastered the skill and trained Dr. Harold Dick and Dr. Leo Scott. They treated thousands and thousands of patients and passed it down to Dr. Bill Carroll (Dr. Otis G. Carroll's son), Dr. Jared Zeff, and Dr. Letitia Dick-Kronenberg (Dr. Harold Dick's daughter). Dr. Zeff and Dr. Dick-Kronenberg have personally kept the method alive by hand-training hundreds of physicians, including ME!

An intolerance is the body's inability to digest and metabolize a food. If digestion is disrupted, then toxemia follows. Toxemia is the root cause of most illnesses, because as taught in naturopathic medical school by our forefathers, there are only three causes to illness:

1. The abnormal composition of blood and lymph

2. Toxemia: The accumulation of morbid matter and waste

3. Decreased vitality

There are a lot of details in the Carroll Method, but it has been observed that most people have some sort of simple food intolerances, usually to a main food group and to a specific combination of foods. The major food intolerances are:

- Potato

- Egg

- Dairy

- Fruit

- Meat

The food combination intolerances are foods that when eaten together, NOT separate of each other, are not digestible and thus not metabolized by a person. The common ones are:

- ⊘ Fruit and sugar

- ⊘ Fruit and grain

- ⊘ Grain and sugar

- ⊘ Potato and grain

- ⊘ Potato and sugar

It has been observed that if you separate these combinations by a certain number of hours, then you can eat them both, but not together at the same time.

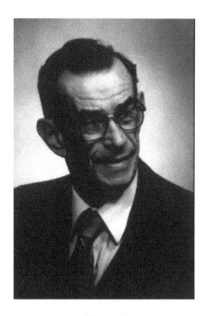

Harold Dick, ND

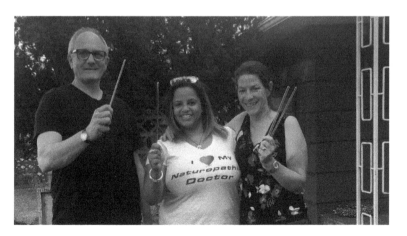

Dr. Jared Zeff, Me, and Dr. Letitia Dick-Kronenberg

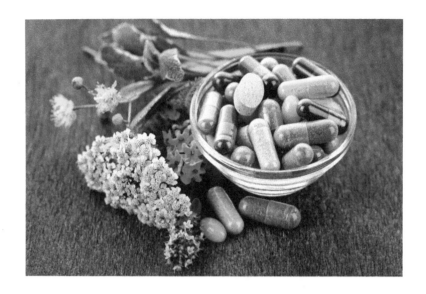

Supplements

I most definitely think that you can use food as your medicine, especially food that you grow, buy at a farmer's market,
and shop for around the perimeter of the grocery store. This
is fresh produce—live and viable food full of nutrients. Our
soil is depleted of lots of the vitamins and minerals that it used
to have back in our great grandparents' day and age, and I
believe that this contributes to some (not all) of our ailments
that we see today. Until you can regulate your diet to a genet-
ic-based customized diet, you will need to supplement with
the things that are lacking. When your body is lacking certain
vitamins, minerals, and nutrients, we call this a "deficiency."

Just as a depletion of vitamins, minerals, and nutrients can cause ailments, so can an excess. Both an excess and deficiency of these nutrients can be corrected with proper diet to an extent, but it definitely takes time, effort, and research to make sure you are doing it correctly.

Many of my patients are in pain. They are tired, and we need to find solutions that will work faster than just changing the diet alone. This is where supplements in the form of herbs, vitamins, minerals, and amino acids come into the mix. Please note that in order to really make a change, we must change your milieu (the intricate balance of how your body works), which in essence means a lifestyle change for most people. As experts in natural medicine, naturopathic physicians are also trained to know the mechanisms of actions of the vitamins, minerals, herbs, amino acids, and homeopathy to help you get the best reaction possible and to guide you in your journey toward optimal health. With that being said, let's talk about supplements.

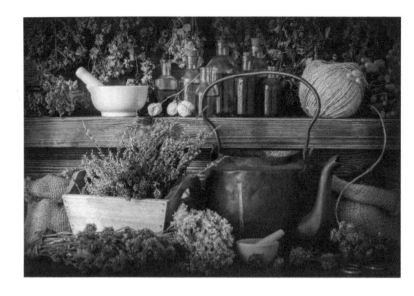

A. Herbs (Tea and Tincture)

Herbs or botanicals are powerful and medicinal. Did you know that most prescription drugs are derived from a plant? The pharmaceutical companies know that the botanical extract works in a certain way, so they study it, extract the main constituent, and then compound it into a synthetic form to market and sell back to you at exorbitant prices. A perfect example are statin drugs. Statin drugs came from a plant called red yeast rice. Red yeast rice is a Chinese culinary ingredient that contains monacolin K (the active constituent that has been studied to lower cholesterol levels). Once the drug companies caught on, they found a way to extract this constituent, and it is now labeled as lovastatin. Sound familiar? Please do not be fooled into thinking that red yeast rice does not have side effects. It does. It has the same side effects as a statin drug, and thus should never be taken unless under the supervision of a naturopathic physician or other licensed health care provider trained in botanicals and natural medicine. The main side effect is rhabdomyolysis (a condition in which muscle fibers break down, releasing substances that can harm the kidneys into the bloodstream). As experts in natural medicine, we know these side effects and know how to use natural medicine to account for them or mitigate them. I always use CoQ10 when giving red yeast rice or when patients come to me taking a statin drug. CoQ10 can be given in a pill form and acts as a natural antioxidant (a substance used to protect the body from damage). It is used to create energy in the cell, which helps with growth and maintenance.

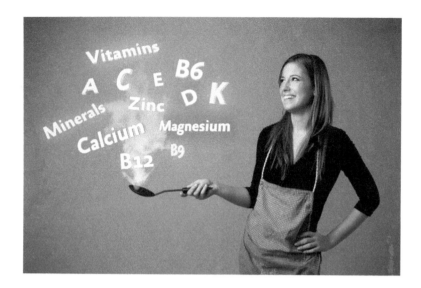

B. Vitamins

The formal definition of a vitamin is "any of a group of organic compounds that are essential for normal growth and nutrition and are required in small quantities in the diet because they cannot be synthesized by the body." There are 13 essential vitamins that your body needs for vital health. They contribute to your vital force; regulate your mood, energy, and beauty (hair, nails, and skin); and even affect the aging process. So yes, they are vital.

1. Vitamin A

Benefits: immunity, bones, teeth, eyes, skin, hair and nails, detox of environmental pollutants

Food sources: carrots, salmon, egg yolks, cold water fish, mango, pink grapefruit, sweet potato

Symptoms if out of balance: macular degeneration and night blindness, cancer, heart disease, stroke, delayed growth in children, rapid aging of skin, dry eyes

2. Vitamin C

Benefits: wound healing; iron absorption; antioxidant; laxative; strengthening gums, teeth, bone, collagen, and connective tissue

Food sources: papaya, cabbage, citrus fruits, berries, vegetables, strawberries, red and green bell pepper, broccoli

Symptoms if out of balance: asthma, common cold, scurvy, diabetes, hypertension, muscle weakness, easy bruising, cancer,

Overdose: diarrhea

3. Vitamin D

Benefits: bones, mood

Food sources: fortified milk, soy/rice drinks, butter, egg yolks, dandelion root, lemongrass, garlic

Symptoms if out of balance: depression, renal/kidney and heart damage

4. Vitamin E

Benefits: antioxidant, muscles, lactation, cancer prevention, reproduction, wounds, prevents blood clots

Food sources: eggs, nuts (almonds), margarine, seeds, vegetable oils, olives, green leafy vegetables, brown rice, wheat germ, corn

Symptoms if out of balance: common cold, low birth weight babies, nerve abnormalities

5. Vitamin K

Benefits: prevents blood clotting, osteoporosis, and menstrual disorders; regulates blood sugar

Food sources: broccoli, eggs, chicken liver, leafy greens (kale, collards, spinach, turnips, mustards), lettuce, Brussel sprouts

Symptoms if out of balance: menstrual pain and excess bleeding, nausea and vomiting in pregnancy, osteoporosis, blood clotting dysfunction, and jaundice in infants

These first five are fat soluble, meaning that they travel through the lymphatic system of the small intestines and are eventually stored in the liver or fat tissue.

The following eight are water soluble, which means they are excreted via urine. This is why you may see a change in color when taking your vitamins. Therefore, they need to be replaced more frequently. I refer to these as the "Mighty Bs." I suggest always taking these with food, as taking them without may cause nausea in some people.

6. Vitamin B1- Thiamine

Benefits: nerves, appetite, digestion, energy metabolism, fertility, lactation, concentration

Food sources: legumes, nuts, seeds, kelp, dates, garlic, wild rice, parsley, watercress, wheatgrass

Symptoms if out of balance: anxiety, depression, hysteria, beriberi (in alcoholics), loss of appetite, muscle cramps

7. Vitamin B2- Riboflavin

Benefits: adrenal function; healthy skin, nails and hair; vision

Food sources: lean meat, mushrooms, poultry, apricot, apple, dates, figs, garlic, kelp, mushrooms, spinach, parsley

Symptoms if out of balance: vision problems, sores/cracks around the mouth and nose

8. Vitamin B3- Niacin

Benefits: lowers cholesterol

Food sources: seafood, lean meats, poultry, legumes, peanuts, tuna, bran, almonds, alfalfa, apricots, chamomile, figs, and garlic

Symptoms if out of balance: pellagra (characterized by dermatitis, diarrhea, mouth sores, dementia),

Overdose: hot flashes, ulcers, high blood sugar, cardiac arrhythmia, uric acid (gout)

9.   Vitamin B5- Pantothenic Acid

Benefits: normalizes red blood cells, lowers cholesterol, regulates hormones, regulates blood sugar levels

Food sources: nuts (almonds and walnuts), alfalfa, meat sources, oranges, peas, seeds, oats, soybeans, broccoli, avocado, legumes

Symptoms if out of balance: adrenal fatigue

10. Vitamin B6- Pyridoxine

Benefits: metabolism of proteins and carbohydrates; nerves and red blood cell;, balances sodium, potassium and phosphorus; skin, teeth, muscles

Food sources: meat, fish, poultry, bananas, green leafy vegetables, potatoes, soybeans, bananas, broccoli, bell pepper, beets, lemon, peas, sprouts, cantaloupe

Symptoms if out of balance: irritability, convulsions, itchy/scaling skin, nerve damage

11. Vitamin B7- Biotin

Benefits: energy, healthy skin and hair, weight loss, healthy blood sugar levels, heart

Food sources: spinach, cauliflower, broccoli, bananas, potatoes, egg yolks, kidney and liver meat, nuts, yeast, cheese, peanut butter, alfalfa

Symptoms if out of balance: dry scalp, dandruff, hair loss (baldness), fatigue, loss of appetite, pain, depression

12. Vitamin B9- Folate (NOT Folic Acid)

Benefits: mental/emotional (brain function), muscles, red blood cells

Food sources: oranges, avocado, spinach, asparagus, legumes, parsley, tomato, cantaloupe, asparagus, organ meats

Symptoms if out of balance: cancer, heart disease, anxiety, depression, infertility, neural tube defects, GI upset (diarrhea), anemia

Overdose: convulsions

13. Vitamin B12

Benefits: nerves (myelin and growth), red blood cells, concentration and memory

Food sources: Certain types of fish, meat, eggs, milk, cheese, liver, kelp, nuts, seeds, garlic, alfalfa

Symptoms if out of balance: fatigue, weakness, megaloblastic anemia, pernicious anemia

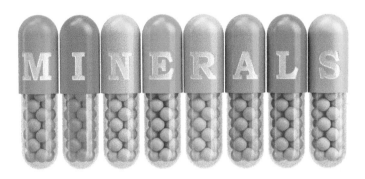

C. Minerals

There are 14 minerals that are sometimes broken down into macro and trace. Trace minerals are termed this because they are only needed in "trace" or small amounts (less than 20mg/day). The trace minerals are iron, manganese, zinc, copper, fluoride, molybdenum, iodine, chromium, and selenium. The macro or major minerals are those that our body needs in large quantities. They are calcium, potassium, magnesium, chloride, sulphur, and phosphorus. Both forms are necessary to maintain life, as they help maintain water balance, metabolism, and bone health through hormone production, nerve conduction, and muscle contractions. All are critical for the body to function optimally, and we cannot say that one is more necessary than the other. Let's take a deeper look at them individually.

1. Calcium

Benefits: energy, nerves, bones/teeth, blood clotting, insomnia, menopause, obesity, blood pressure, electrolyte

Food sources: broccoli, turnip greens, dairy products (cheese, milk, yogurt), nuts, canned salmon, sardines, seeds, leafy green vegetables (spinach), orange juice, cereals, oysters, rice beverages, soy, almonds, black-eyed peas, green peas

Symptoms if out of balance: hypertension, sleep issues, dental health issues, PMS, osteoporosis, kidney stones

2. Magnesium

Benefits: enzyme activity and energy, prevents birth defects, muscle relaxer, improves sleep, prevents constipation, decreases anxiety and stress, electrolyte

Food sources: dairy, fish, leafy greens, meat, molasses, seafood, seeds, soybeans, tomatoes, beet greens, broad beans, lima beans, artichokes, sweet potatoes, buckwheat flour, pumpkin seeds, peanuts, wheat flour, oat bran, barley, cornmeal, chocolate

Symptoms if out of balance: chronic fatigue, depression, insomnia, PMS, anxiety, cramps, diabetes, heart attack, constipation, migraines, nausea, irritability, muscle weakness, twitching, cardiac arrhythmia

Overdose: nausea, vomiting, low blood pressure, nervous system disorders

3. Iodine

Benefits: thyroid, metabolism, flushes toxins

Food sources: Iodized salt, kelp, dulse, shellfish, deep-water whitefish (cod, haddock, halibut, herring perch, salmon, sea bass), brown seaweed, canned sardines, tuna, lobster, oyster, spinach, turnip greens, clams, shrimp garlic, lima beans, Swiss chard, squash, sesame seeds, soybeans

Symptoms if out of balance: fibrocystic breast disease, goiter, skin conditions, hormonal imbalances

4. Selenium

Benefits: anti-cancer, antioxidant, thyroid, bone growth, immune system, anti-inflammatory

Food sources: Brazil nuts, brewer's/torula yeast, brown rice, meat (animal kidneys), seafood (fish, tuna, crabs, and lobsters), whole grains, mushrooms, eggs

Symptoms if out of balance: hypothyroidism, weight gain, fatigue, fungal and microbial infections, hair loss, dandruff, rheumatoid arthritis, gout, eczema

5. Zinc

Benefits: immune system, reproduction, skin care, weight loss, smell/taste/vision, bones

Food sources: eggs, legumes, seafood (oysters, shrimp, crab), whole grains, beef, turkey, whole grains, peanuts

Symptoms if out of balance: common cold, acne, eczema, night blindness, fungal infections, hair loss (alopecia), acne, prostate issues, slow healing of wounds, loss of taste, retarded growth, delayed sexual development in children

Overdose: nausea, vomiting, diarrhea, abdominal pain, gastric bleeding

6. Chromium

Benefits: energy, sugar metabolism

Food sources: beef, brewer's yeast, brown rice, meat, whole grains, beets, cardamom, cloves, dulse, garlic, kelp, mushrooms, wheatgrass, onions

Symptoms if out of balance: diabetes, glucose intolerance, insulin resistance, hyperglycemia, weight changes

7. Copper

Benefits: builds blood cells, bone, collagen, circulatory system, brain, hair

Food sources: oysters, whole grains (wheat bran, oats), meat (liver), seafood, beans, soy flour and soy beans, avocados, barley, garlic, nuts (almonds), blackstrap molasses, beets, lentils, copper pipes, copper cookware

Symptoms if out of balance: throat infection, arthritis, hemoglobin deficiency, grey hair, anemia that is unresponsive to iron therapy

Overdose: liver disease, vomiting, diarrhea

8. Manganese

Benefits: fat and protein metabolism, energy, sugar levels, thyroid, digestion, wound healing

Food sources: avocados, nuts, seeds, green vegetables, brown rice, coconuts, almonds, hazelnuts, sea vegetables, raspberries, pineapples, garlic, grapes, beetroot, green beans, rice, peppermint, oats, watercress, mustard greens, strawberries, blackberries, tropical fruits, lettuce, spinach, molasses, cloves, turmeric, leeks, tofu, whole wheat, bananas, cucumbers, kiwis, figs, carrots

Symptoms if out of balance: fatigue, osteoporosis, epilepsy, inflammation, sprains, PMS, sprains

9. Phosphorus

Benefits: muscles, bones, brain, digestion, balance of hormones, stimulates riboflavin and niacin

Food sources: meat (chicken breast), nuts, legumes, dairy products (milk, egg yolks, cheese), sunflower seeds, rice, white bread, potatoes, broccoli, peas, lentils, peanut butter, tuna, pork, soda beverages

Symptoms if out of balance: muscle weakness, sexual weakness, stunted growth, tremors, numbness, anxiety, loss of appetite, tooth decay, and bone pain. (Most people suffering from anorexia have dangerously low levels of phosphorous.)

10. Potassium

Benefits: lowers blood pressure, blood sugar regulation, boosts brain function, optimal nerve and brain function, optimal fluid balance, electrolyte

Food sources: fish (salmon), whole grains, citrus fruits, vegetables (broccoli, green beans), chicken, whole milk, fresh fruit juices (orange), almonds, nuts, lima beans, potatoes, avocados, bananas, coconut water, peanuts, bananas, oranges, sunflower seeds

Symptoms if out of balance: diabetes, mental fog, arthritis, kidney disorder, anxiety/stress, heart palpitations or irregular heartbeat, severe headaches, anemia, fatigue, muscle weakness, nausea, anorexia, irritability

11. Silicon

Benefits: collagen for bones and connective tissues, sleep, skin, prevents aluminum toxicity, nails, prevents insomnia

Food sources: alfalfa, bell pepper, brown rice, root vegetables, soy, horsetail, apples, cereals, raw cabbage, peanuts, carrots, onions, cucumber, pumpkin, fish, unrefined grains, oats, almonds, oranges

Symptoms if out of balance: sleep issues, skin issues (wrinkles), brittle nails, thinning hair (alopecia)

12. Sodium

Benefits: water balance, prevents sunstroke, brain function, regulates sugar, skin, electrolyte

Food sources: apples, common salt, homemade soups, cabbage, egg yolks, pulses, bananas, carrots, baking powder and baking soda, turnips, leafy vegetables, dried peas

Symptoms if out of balance: muscle cramps, confusion, exhaustion, headache, diarrhea, weight loss, low blood pressure

13. Iron

Benefits: blood cells, growth, immune system, energy

Food sources: eggs, fish, liver, meat, leafy vegetables, whole grains

Symptoms if out of balance: anemia, muscle weakness, GI disorders, restless leg syndrome, skin pallor, fatigue, headaches, shortness of breath, difficulty concentrating, brittle nails, cracked lips

Overdose: constipation

14. Boron

Benefits: bone, brain, sexual function, anti-aging, muscle pain

Food sources: fruit (apples, oranges, red grapes, pears, plums, kiwis, sultanas, dates, currants), vegetables (avocado, soybeans), nuts (hazelnuts), chickpeas, borlotti beans, peanut butter, red kidney beans, tomato, lentils, olive, onion, potato wine, and beer

Symptoms if out of balance: strokes, heart attacks, rheumatoid arthritis, postmenopausal osteoporosis, blood clots

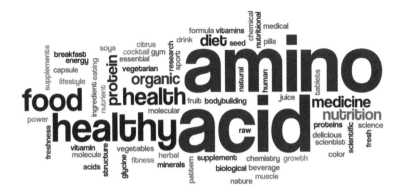

D. Amino Acids

There are a total of 20 amino acids. Nine are considered essential, and the other 11 are non-essential. The essential ones must be consumed through our diet because our body does not make them. They are histidine, leucine, isoleucine, lysine, methionine, phenylalanine, threonine, tryptophan, and valine. The 11 non-essentials are made naturally by our body. They are alanine, asparagine, aspartic acid, cysteine, glutamic acid, glutamine, glycine, proline, serine, and tyrosine

Amino acids are the building blocks of protein in our body. They help eliminate excess fat stored in the bloodstream and help to stimulate metabolism and energy production. They often are precursors to another molecule.

An amino acid deficiency could be the reason for your lack of mental alertness, changes in skin or hair color, reproduction issues, and other health issues. Let's take a closer look at the nine essentials.

1. Histidine

Benefits: helps protect tissues from damage caused by radiation and heavy metals, benefits mental and physical health through the myelin sheath that transmits messages between the brain and the organs.

Food sources: beef, lamb, cheese, pork, chicken, turkey, soy, fish, nuts, seeds, eggs, beans, whole grains

Symptoms if out of balance: rheumatoid arthritis, allergic reactions, ulcers, anemia caused by kidney failure or kidney dialysis, anxiety, schizophrenia

2. Leucine

Benefits: builds muscle, provides energy, muscle recovery, helps with muscle wasting

Food sources: meats (fish, chicken, turkey), dairy products (yogurt and cheese), soybeans, eggs, nuts, seeds, and fruit

Symptoms if out of balance: kidney issues from a buildup of ammonia, hypoglycemia, GI distress, and pellagra (niacin deficiency)

3. Isoleucine

Benefits: regulates energy, blood sugar, and formation of hemoglobin. As a supplement, it helps with physical endurance and healing and repair of muscular tissue.

Food sources: nuts, seeds, all meats, chickpeas, lentils, fish, eggs, soy

Symptoms if out of balance: hypoglycemia

4. Lysine

Benefits: A natural disease-fighting agent, decrease outbreaks of Herpes Simplex Virus, prevents anxiety, prevents diarrhea, increases the absorption of calcium, reduces diabetes-related problems, healthy GI

Food sources: beans, yogurt, animal proteins

Symptoms if out of balance: anemia, apathy, bloodshot eyes, depression, edema, fatigue, fever blisters, hair loss, inability to concentrate, infertility, irritability, lethargy, liver damage, loss of energy, muscle loss, retarded growth, stomach ulcers, weakness

5. Methionine

Benefits: prevents liver damage if you overdose on Tylenol; production of collagen to enhance the condition of skin, hair, and nails; boosts the immune system; produces SAMe (S-Adenosyl-L-methionine), which is used to treat psychiatric ill-nesses, infertility, liver problems, premenstrual disorders, and musculoskeletal conditions

Food sources: meat, fish, and dairy products

Symptoms if out of balance: autoimmune disease, liver de-toxification problems, heavy metal toxicity, depression, anxi-ety, seizures, ADD, ADHD, cardiovascular disease

6. Phenylalanine

Benefits: precursor to another amino acid in the production of neurotransmitters that affect mood; production of melanin by the skin

Food sources: beef, chicken, pork, fish, milk, yogurt, eggs, cheese, soybeans, tofu, some nuts, seeds, and legumes

Symptoms is out of balance: confusion, decreased alertness, faulty memory, depression, sluggish metabolism, lack of en-ergy, reduced appetite, vitiligo (due to not enough melanin production)

7. Threonine

Benefits:

➲ Cardiovascular: Keeps connective tissues and muscles throughout the body, including the heart, strong and elastic

- ◉ Liver: Digestion of fats and fatty acids. Without it, fats would build up in the liver and cause liver failure

- ◉ Central nervous and immune system function: Aids in the production of antibodies which has been helpful with ALS, MS, and depression

Food sources: dairy foods, meat, grains, mushrooms, leafy vegetables

Symptoms is out of balance: emotional agitation, confusion, digestion difficulties, fatty liver

8. Tryptophan

Benefits: helps with depression, anxiety, and insomnia; weight loss; decreases cholesterol

Food sources: fish, egg, milk, chocolate, spirulina

Symptoms is out of balance: confusion, anxiety, muscle weakness, incoordination

9. Valine

Benefits: blood sugar regulation, normal growth, tissue repair, proper mental functioning, stimulation of the CNS, energy

Food sources: meats, dairy products, mushrooms, peanuts, soy protein

Symptoms is out of balance: fatty liver, leukopenia, hypoalbuminemia, hair loss, unwanted weight loss

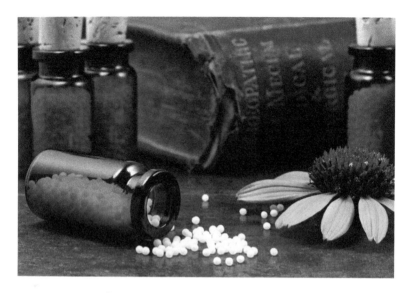

E. Homeopathy

Homeopathy is also a key in healing the sick. While it is quite complicated to explain (at least for me) if you have never experienced it yourself, your naturopathic physician will do a very detailed questionnaire and ask questions that no one else has ever asked you. Such questions could include whether you prefer to sit in the shade or the sun, whether you prefer salt or sweets, or whether you stick one foot out of the covers when you are lying in bed.

I enlisted the help of a great friend, classmate and colleague to help better explain homeopathy. Dr. Eli Camp is a licensed naturopathic physician and is board certified in homeopathy.

She is also the co-author of *The Unvaccinated Child: A Treatment Guide for Parents and Caregivers.*

Here is her explanation:

> When it comes to stimulating your innate healing ability, one of the safest and most effective therapies is homeopathy. Used by doctors for more then 200 years, this therapy is based on a healing principle called "like cures like." The medicines used in this therapy are called homeopathic remedies and they are prepared by diluting a substance to incredibly small amounts. They are so dilute that one has to have very special equipment to detect any of the physical molecules of the original substance. And in fact, it is this dilution that makes homeopathy so safe!

> It is natural to ask, if there are so few molecules, how could it possibly do anything in the body? Even though the remedies are diluted and carry few molecules of the original medicine, they do carry the *information* from the original substance. It is this information that your body uses to help correct the underlying imbalance that has led to symptoms of illness.

> This has been the choice of treatment by many highly educated people, royalty, world leaders, the general public, major athletes, and more. Homeopathy is so safe there are no contraindications. It is also very affordable; most remedies cost about $10. It can be used at any age and can

treat things from the simple cold to more complex and chronic illness.

F.   Cell Salts

Dr. Wilhelm Schuessler, a German doctor, founded the use of biochemical cell salt therapy in 1873. These mineral cell salts satisfy mineral imbalances. Dr. Schuessler said that "deficiencies in these minerals are the source of common health problems, and the cell salts derived from these minerals give the body what it needs to treat illness and be well." Dr. Schuessler combined the principles of biochemistry with homeopathy to give us the 12 safe and natural cell salts, each derived from one of the 12 inorganic mineral compounds most important to our cellular health.

Here is a very brief explanation of each:

#1 CALC. FLUOR.	#2 CALC. PHOS.	#3 CALC. SULPH.	#4 FERRUM PHOS.	#5 KALI MUR.	#6 KALI PHOS.
Colds, Hemorrhoids, Chapped Skin	Teething, Sore Throat	Colds, Sore Throat, Acne	Fevers, Minor Swelling, Colds	Colds, Sore Throat, Runny Nose	Stress, Simple Nervous Tension, Headaches
#7 KALI SULPH.	#8 MAG. PHOS.	#9 NAT. MUR.	#10 NAT. PHOS.	#11 NAT. SULPH.	#12 SILICEA
Colds, Skin Eruptions	Muscle Cramps and Pains	Headaches, Colds, Heartburn, Gastric Upset and Distress	Indigestion, Gas, Hyperacidity	Flu, Nausea, Vomiting	Skin Eruptions, Brittle Hair and Nails

Bioplasma	A combination of all twelve cell salts to support cellular health and function		Biochemic Phosphates	Nervous Exhaustion, Irritability, and Sleeplessness

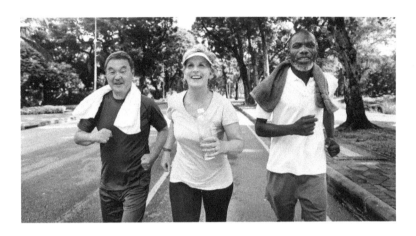

Movement

Most people do not want to hear about exercising, especially when their time is limited. Let's call it physical activity. Physical activity can be exercise if you want, but it could also be dancing or golfing with a friend. Regular physical activity or exercise can increase your quality of life by decreasing your risk factor for certain adverse events like heart attack and type 2 diabetes. Physical activity can increase your stamina, which lets you use less energy for the same amount of work, thus increasing your energy for things that are fun, like running around with your kids or grandkids.

Exercise works on both physical and mental well-being. Physical activity decreases stress, lifts your mood, and allows you to sleep better.

There are five areas that are connected to movement in which structural alignment is so crucial to get blood flow, life force, muscles, and bones in the correct position. This can be accomplished with Naturopathic Manipulative Therapies (NMT), Osteopathic Manipulative Therapies (OMT), chiropractic adjustment, and massage therapy. Let me list them for you.

A. Cranial Sacral or Cranial Osteopathy

    ⊙ Done by a naturopathic physician, DO, chiropractor, or massage therapist. This is a very gentle manipulation of your cranial bones and is amazing for headaches, migraines, and TMJ.

B. Lymphatic Massage

    ⊙ Typically done by a massage therapist or physical therapist who is specifically trained to stimulate the lymph system through light touch and smooth motions

    ⊙ Remove toxins, increase circulation, and dump accumulated waste

C. Skeletal Adjustment

    ⊙ Done by a naturopathic physician, DO, or chiropractor

    ⊙ Manipulation helps to optimize the nervous system

Chiropractic is a field that primarily focuses on the musculoskelatal system and the nervous system. These two systems are deeply intertwined and have had a tremendous effect on your health and well-being. Chiropractors utilize a natural, hands-on approach to your health to get you moving better and ultimately feeling better. Chiropractors are highly trained in diagnosing and treating a wide-range of conditions and incorporate a variety of treatment options including manipulation/adjustment, therapeutic exercise, and nutritional/lifestyle counseling.

Shane MacPhee, DC

D. Connective Tissue (Ligaments/Meniscus) Adjustments, Ultrasound, and Massage

➲ Done by a naturopathic physician, doctor of osteopathic medicine, chiropractor, or massage therapist.

E. Muscle

➲ Adjustments of the skeletal axis relax the muscle. The best things would be to get an adjustment and then follow up with a massage.

Described below are specific movements that are effective for each blood type.

EXERCISE REGIMEN for Blood Type O

Intense Physical Exercises:

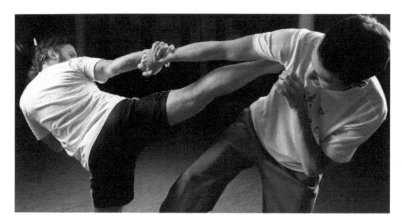

Martial Arts

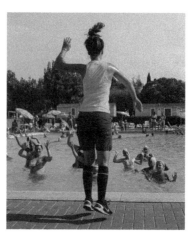

Aerobics

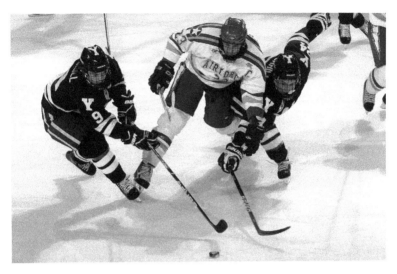

Contact Sports

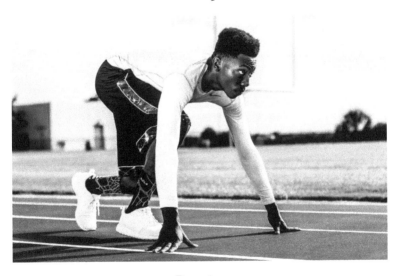

Running

EXERCISE REGIMEN *for Blood Type A*

Calming Exercises:

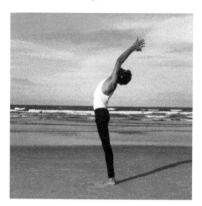

Yoga

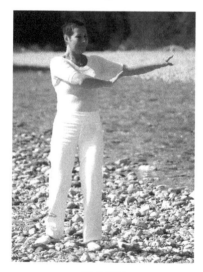

Tai Chi

EXERCISE REGIMEN for Blood Type B

Moderate physical with mental balance:

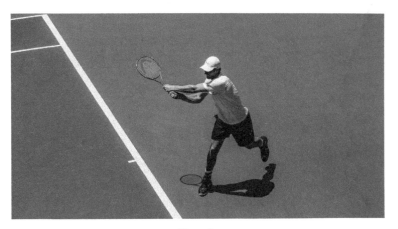

Tennis

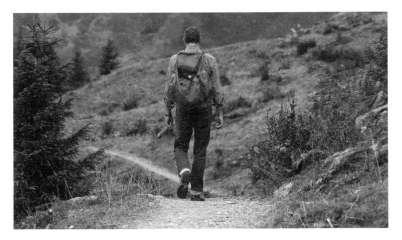

Hiking

Exercise Regimen for Blood Type B Continued

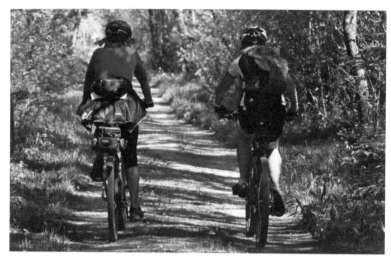

Cycling

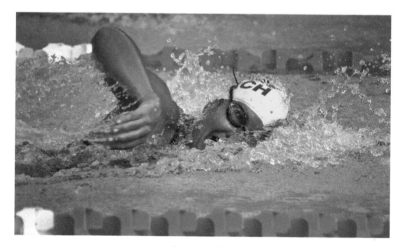

Swimming

EXERCISE REGIMEN for Blood Type AB

Calming Exercises

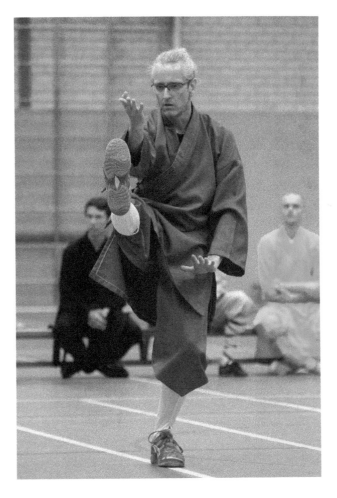

Tai Chi

Exercise Regimen for Blood Type AB Continued

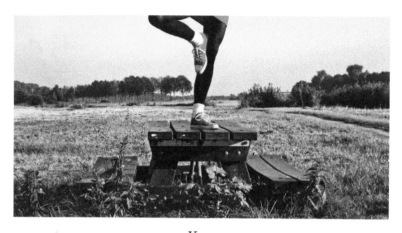

Yoga

Moderate physical

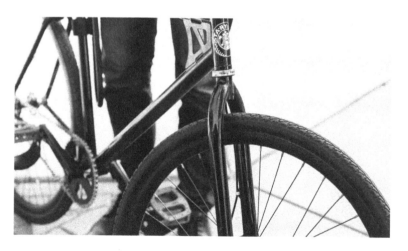

Cycling

Exercise Regimen for Blood Type AB Continued

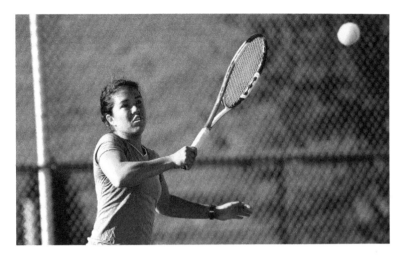

Tennis

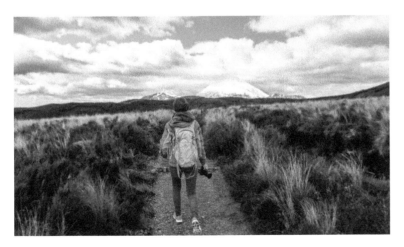

Hiking

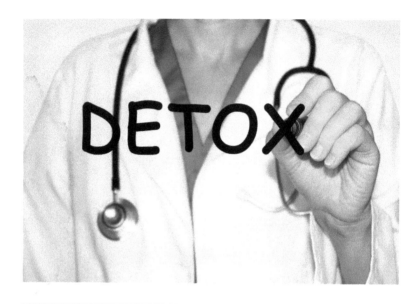

Detox

Absolutely everything that I have previously talked about falls into this category. Your thoughts can be toxic, and so can your emotions, so I consider positive thoughts an emotional detox. Lack of sleep can be toxic in that you are not allowing your body to heal itself, so sleeping properly is considered a detox. The proper use of water and your choices of how to drink it and use it can be a detox. Proper alignment of the body eliminates inflammation in our joints and muscles, which is a detox for our skeletal system. With all the pollution in the air, the non-fertile soil in which our food is grown, our pesticide-laced foods that we eat, and all the negativity that surrounds us, we need to do daily detoxes. Everything mentioned up until this point can be used as a daily detox. The following are my top six secrets for daily detoxing.

A. Food Choices

This is top on the list, as it affects so many of the others. You must eat food, so choose foods that are not inflammatory for your genetics. Follow a customized diet based on your genetics or simply follow the blood type diet. There are herbs that we know specifically help to detox certain organs and can be used quite successfully. Herbs are food, and this is why they are included in this section. It is always my suggestion that you consult with a naturopathic physician before you start using herbs. May I please share with you some examples of detoxing herbs? I thought you might say yes, so here are some of the greats.

	Black Walnut Hull	Parasite/Anti fungal
	Blue Vervain	Relax nerves, Blood cleanser
	Cascara Powder	Purgative (cleans colon)
	Clove	Parasite cleansing

	Dandelion Root	Kidney stones, blood cleanser
	Elderberry	Mucus detox, cold, flu
	Gentian	Improves digestion and treats a number of GI complaints
	Guaco	Blood cleanser
	Kelp	Heavy metal detox, chemo detox, iodine
	Lilly of the Valley	Heart herb, dissolves kidney stones
	Milk Thistle	Cancer, liver detox
	Mullein	Mucus detox, asthma
	Poke Root	Cleans lymphatic system, endometriosis

	Prodgiosa	Purgative (colon cleanser)
	Rhubarb Root Powder	Purgative (colon cleanse)
	Sarsaparilla root	High iron, anemia, sickle cell
	Uva Ursi	Weight loss, increase Kidney function
	Wormwood	Parasites
	Yellowdock Root	High iron content, anemia, sickle cell

B. Poop

You will read about the importance of pooping all the time if you follow my blogs or read my books. You will hear it all the time if you listen to my podcasts, watch Facebook live videos, attend any function at which I am speaking, and especially if you are a #VitalONE (one of my special concierge patients). Proper digestion of our food is a key component or secret to health. If you are digesting the food that you eat well, then you are also able to eliminate the waste or portion that you do not need. Part of digestion is to use the food for fuel and also be able to burn off the toxins and excrete the waste. Proper bowel movements (2-3 times a day) ensure that we do not have a buildup of waste and toxins floating around our body. If you are not pooping at least once a day, there is a problem, and we would consider this constipation. Ideally, you should be pooping 30 minutes to an hour after each meal (not snack). Go back to my infant example. How many times do you change an infant's poopy diaper? Pretty much each time they eat, right? This should be true for adults as well.

Type 1 and 2: Constipation. Difficult to pass and require straining.

Type 3: Healthy. Slides out easily without foul odor or marks. Typical of a healthy vegetarian diet.

Type 4: Healthy. Slides out easily without foul odor or marks. Typical of a healthy diet with animal protein.

Type 5: Precursor to diarrhea. Re-evaluate your diet. Reduce fruit intake, cut out alcohol and processed foods, and try to balance the animal protein, veggies, and grains.

Type 6 and 7: Diarrhea. Difficult to control. The body is unable to extract water, electrolytes, and nutrients from the food, causing malnourishment and dehydration.

BRISTOL STOOL CHART

	Type 1	Separate hard lumps	**SEVERE CONSTIPATION**
	Type 2	Lumpy and sausage like	**MILD CONSTIPATION**
	Type 3	A sausage shape with cracks in the surface	**NORMAL**
	Type 4	Like a smooth, soft sausage or snake	**NORMAL**
	Type 5	Soft blobs with clear-cut edges	**LACKING FIBER**
	Type 6	Mushy consistency with ragged edges	**MILD DIARRHEA**
	Type 7	Liquid consistency with no solid pieces	**SEVERE DIARRHEA**

Photo Credit: Wikipedia

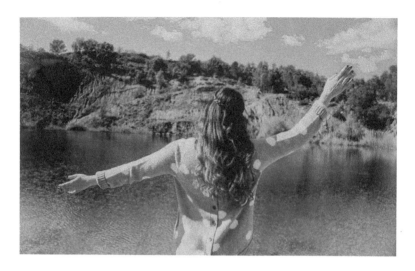

C. Fresh Air

Air is important, as it brings and sustains life. Each cell in our body requires oxygen. Our heart needs it to beat, our muscles need it to function and move properly, our lungs need it so that we can breathe, and our brain needs it so that we can think clearly and articulate thoughts. Air, along with water, is one of those essential things needed to sustain life. When a loved one is put on life support, they are essentially being given air/oxygen to circulate to cells within their body to keep them alive. Many times, this works and allows the body to heal. Fresh air is God given and abundant. It does the body and the soul good.

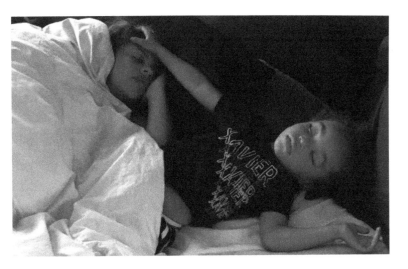

My son and I asleep—my favorite pastime

D. Proper Sleep

One of my top priorities for patients is that they must get proper sleep and the proper amount of sleep. Proper sleep is when you go into REM (rapid eye movement). This signifies that you are in restorative and restful sleep. This is the time when your body heals itself. Your body's immune system comes alive during restful sleep and starts working like a doctor to heal the minor tears, aches and pains, cells that replicated the wrong way (cancer), and any other minor detail that is not just the way God intended it to be. The master hormone of the immune system is melatonin. Many of you who have insomnia have tried melatonin as a supplement to help you sleep with great success. Our body makes melatonin naturally. Instead of taking a supplement, why not just get the proper sleep and the proper amount of it? Melatonin is made in the body between 10pm and 2am. This is why I do not get text messages from patients between these hours—because they should all be asleep. Right, Vital Ones? The last step to establish your restful sleep is to determine the proper amount of sleep. Everyone has heard that you should get eight hours of sleep daily. Well, I beg to differ. I believe that the amount of sleep needed for rejuvenation is individualized. I personally need nine to ten hours of sleep, but my husband is refreshed with just six hours. Regardless of the number of hours that you sleep, there are three main points.

1.   Four of the hours need to be between 10pm and 2am.

2.   Did you get into REM?

3.   When you woke up, did you feel refreshed?

If you accomplish the above three points, then you are doing a daily detox each time you sleep.

E.   Tea

My love for tea was born well before me. My mom never drank coffee. She is a tea connoisseur. She starts her day with tea and usually ends it with tea as well. She likes black tea with lemon and sugar, especially as the first cup of the day. I prefer green tea due to all the medicinal benefits. I love the fact that there are so many different teas to choose from and that

I will never get bored from lack of flavors or choice. What is really exciting is that most teas are herbs and have some type of medicinal benefits. Yes, tea can be a medicine! I often give my family elderberry tea or an Echinacea tea if they appear to have the symptoms of a cold. In fact, sometimes I give it as a prophylactic due to the season or if I know something is going around. If someone has an uncomfortable belly ache from overeating, I will give spearmint or peppermint. If someone is nauseated, I will give ginger tea. If they have a headache, I will give peppermint. Tea is simply a hot drink made by infusing the dried, crushed leaves of the tea plant in boiling water. I mentioned several detoxing herbs in the food section that could actually be steeped into a tea. It is always my suggestion that you consult with a naturopathic physician before you start using them.

	Alma Berry	Infertility in males
	Bitter Melon	Diabetes Management
	Bladderwrack	UNDER active thyroid, regulate bowel movements
	Bugleweed	OVERactive thyroid

	Burdock Root	Hair, kidney, blood
	Catnip	Stomach issues, helps onset woman's cycle
	Chaste Tree Berry	PCOS, women issues
	Chickweed	weight loss, urinary issues
	Damiana	Fertility, increases sex drive
	Eyebright	Eye issues
	Feverfew	Migraines
	Hydrangea	Helps urinary issues, prostate
	Irish sea moss	Provides 98% of minerals body needs
	Lemon Verbena	Weight Loss, build muscles, helps calm nerves

	Linden	High blood pressure
	Nopal Cactus	Cholesterol
	Pau D'arco	Pain and inflammation
	Raspberry Leap	PMS, nausea, iron
	Red clover	PMS, cancer (breast) high cholesterol, lung issues
	Rhubarb Root Powder	purgative (colon cleanse)
	Sarsaparilla Root	High iron, anemia, sickle cell
	Valerian Root	Sleep, muscle issues
	Yellow Dock root	High iron content, anemia, sickle cell

I would much rather sip a cup of tea and know that I am healing myself than take a handful of pills, get an IV, or even have surgery. Having alternatives really is great!

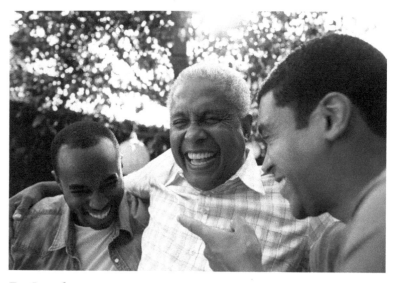

F. Laughter

Laughter is an underrated and underutilized therapy. Laughter secretes "feel-good hormones" and a host of other beneficial substances every time we laugh heartily for extended periods. Laughter also diminishes cortisol (a stress hormone) while increasing immune reactivity. I consider laughter an emotional detox. Cancer Centers of America (CTCA) actually promotes laughter therapy for their patients and has a therapist to moderate the session. My prescription to my patients is 20-30 minutes of roll-on-the-floor, pee-in-your-pants laughter at least once daily. You can talk to a friend, watch a show that makes you laugh, or read a book that is funny. Laughter really is a therapy!

SUMMARY

It all starts with your mindset. What are your thoughts? Try to keep the negative thoughts at bay and replace them with positive ones. Dismiss negative people from your life and surround yourself with positive and encouraging people. Write down your intentions and affirmations and say them daily. Use a gratitude jar or journal to remind yourself of all the things that you are blessed to have and experience. Meditate and pray daily as a daily emotional detox. Treat sleep like a prescription, because it is medicinal and can help boost your immune system and quality of life, especially between 10pm and 2am. Drink half your weight in ounces of fresh, clean, alkalinized water, preferably with electrolytes added.

Start thinking of your food as medicine and/or poison. Learn your blood type and Carroll intolerances and eat accordingly. You have to eat, so why not eat what should make you feel better and give more energy and vitality as opposed to foods that make you tired and upset your stomach? There are lots of supplements to choose from. Some can be helpful and some harmful. Seek out a naturopathic physician to partner with to get the most out of your supplements.

Get your body moving! Exercise correctly according to your blood type and make sure that your structural framework is healthy and aligned by using physical medicine. Last but not least, keep your body clean and healthy by acknowledging that there are possible toxins all around us to which we are exposed daily. Daily detoxing for your mind, body, and spirit will keep you healthy and whole. If you can do even half of these steps on your own, then you are well on your way to a vibrant life. If you need help, I am just a click away at www. DrSammND.com.

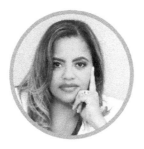

ABOUT THE AUTHOR

Dr. M. Samm Pryce, aka Dr. Samm, is a licensed physician of naturopathic medicine. Passionate about natural healing methods, Dr. Samm's life mission is to guide her patients to live happy, vibrant, and productive lives using simple resources that they already have at their disposal. In particular, Dr. Samm is sought out for her knowledge of the blood type diet and the relationship between epigenetics and nutrigenomics. Currently, Dr. Samm serves as the Chief Medical Officer at Balanced Integration, PLLC. She earned her naturopathic medical degree from Southwest College of Naturopathic Medicine. Following her degree, she rotated through the Family Residency Program at Jamaica Hospital in Jamaica, Queens, New York, and finished the first residency program granted by Dr. Peter D'Adamo at The D'Adamo Clinic in Wilton, Connecticut.

To connect, visit Dr. Samm at www.DrSammND.com

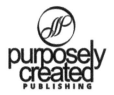

CREATING DISTINCTIVE BOOKS
WITH INTENTIONAL RESULTS

We're a collaborative group of creative masterminds
with a mission to produce high-quality books to position
you for monumental success in the marketplace.

Our professional team of writers, editors, designers,
and marketing strategists work closely together to ensure
that every detail of your book is a clear representation
of the message in your writing.

Want to know more?
Write to us at info@publishyourgift.com
or call (888) 949-6228

Discover great books, exclusive offers, and more at
www.PublishYourGift.com

Connect with us on social media

@publishyourgift

CPSIA information can be obtained
at www.ICGtesting.com
Printed in the USA
LVHW070204240222
711892LV00021B/945

9 781948 400022